Anti Parkinson's Disease Diet Cookbook

Dr. Mary Williams

Disclaimer

Please keep in mind that the content in this book is solely for educational purposes. The information offered here is said to be reliable and trustworthy. The author makes no implication or intends to offer any warranty of accuracy for particular individual cases.

Before beginning any diet or lifestyle habits, it is recommended that you contact a knowledgeable practitioner, such as your doctor. This book's material should not be utilized in place of expert counsel or professional guidance.

The author, publisher, and distributor expressly disclaim all liability, loss, damage, or danger incurred by persons who rely on the information in this book, whether directly or indirectly.

All intellectual property rights are retained. This book's information should not be replicated in any way, mechanically, electronically, photocopying, or by any other methods accessible

Table of Contents

Why You Should Give this Book a Chance

Are you or a loved one navigating the challenges of Parkinson's disease?
Do you seek a holistic approach that not only addresses the symptoms but actively promotes well-being and vitality?

If so, we invite you on a transformative journey with the "Anti Parkinson's Disease Diet Cookbook." Let's explore how these meticulously crafted recipes can be your ally in managing Parkinson's and fostering a life of vitality.

Fuel Your Body with Purpose:
Imagine starting your day with a Berry and Spinach Smoothie that not only tantalizes your taste buds but also floods your system with antioxidants. Antioxidants, found abundantly in berries and leafy greens, are known to combat oxidative stress—a factor linked to Parkinson's disease progression. This cookbook prioritizes ingredients rich in antioxidants, essential for promoting overall brain health.

Harness the Power of Superfoods:
Unlock the potential of Quinoa Porridge with Almonds and Berries, a nutrient-packed powerhouse that goes beyond merely satisfying hunger. Quinoa is a superfood that delivers essential amino acids crucial for neurotransmitter function. Almonds bring healthy fats to the table, supporting cognitive health. These recipes aren't just delicious; they are carefully crafted to nourish your brain.

Every Meal, a Step Toward Wellness:
From Salmon and Avocado Breakfast Wrap to Teriyaki Salmon with Brown Rice, our recipes are meticulously curated to include Omega-3 fatty acids. Research suggests

that Omega-3s may contribute to managing symptoms associated with Parkinson's disease. These dishes are not just culinary delights; they're a strategy for embracing a diet that supports brain health.

Balance and Variety on Your Plate:
Variety is key, and our recipes ensure you savor every moment while supporting your health. The Mediterranean Baked Cod brings together flavors that have been associated with a reduced risk of neurodegenerative diseases. Lentil and Vegetable Curry introduces plant-based protein sources, offering a diverse array of nutrients that your body craves.

Your Comprehensive Guide to a Holistic Lifestyle:
Beyond individual recipes, this cookbook provides a holistic approach, incorporating a wide array of nutrients that play a role in supporting neurological health. From Spinach and Feta Stuffed Chicken Breast, rich in B vitamins, to Pesto Zoodles with Cherry Tomatoes, offering an abundance of essential vitamins and minerals—each dish is a building block in your journey to holistic wellness.

Empower Yourself with Knowledge:
This cookbook isn't just a collection of recipes; it's a gateway to understanding the vital connection between nutrition and neurological health. The detailed nutritional information accompanying each recipe empowers you to make informed choices, allowing you to take charge of your well-being.

Embark on Your Journey Today:
The "Anti Parkinson's Disease Diet Cookbook" is not just a recipe book; it's your companion in the pursuit of a vibrant, healthier life. By exploring the relationship between

nutrition and Parkinson's disease, you're not just cooking; you're engaging in a strategy for well-being. Each recipe is a step toward reclaiming control, embracing balance, and savoring the journey to a healthier you.

Elevate your nutrition. Elevate your life.

RECIPES

Berry and Spinach Smoothie

Intro: This vibrant Berry and Spinach Smoothie is a delicious and nutritious way to kickstart your day. Packed with antioxidants and vitamins, it's a perfect choice for a quick and refreshing breakfast.
Total Prep Time: 5 minutes

Ingredients:
- 1 cup mixed berries (strawberries, blueberries, raspberries)
- 1 cup fresh spinach leaves
- 1 banana
- 1/2 cup Greek yogurt
- 1 tablespoon honey
- 1 cup almond milk
- Ice cubes (optional)

Instructions:
1. Combine all ingredients in a blender.
2. Blend until smooth and creamy.
3. Pour into a glass and enjoy immediately.

Nutritional Information:
Calories: 250 | *Protein:* 12g | *Carbohydrates:* 45g | *Fat:* 5g | *Fiber:* 8g

Quinoa Porridge with Almonds and Berries

Intro: This Quinoa Porridge is a hearty and wholesome alternative to traditional oatmeal. Loaded with protein and fiber, it's a nourishing breakfast that will keep you energized throughout the morning.
Total Prep Time: 20 minutes

Ingredients:
- 1/2 cup quinoa, rinsed
- 1 cup almond milk
- 1/4 teaspoon vanilla extract
- 1/4 cup sliced almonds
- 1/2 cup mixed berries (strawberries, blueberries, blackberries)
- 1 tablespoon honey or maple syrup

Instructions:
1. In a saucepan, combine quinoa and almond milk. Bring to a boil.
2. Reduce heat, cover, and simmer for 15 minutes or until quinoa is cooked.
3. Stir in vanilla extract and top with almonds, berries, and sweetener.
4. Serve warm and enjoy.

Nutritional Information:
Calories: 320 | *Protein:* 10g | *Carbohydrates:* 45g | *Fat:* 12g | *Fiber:* 7g

Avocado Toast with Poached Egg

Intro: Avocado Toast with a perfectly poached egg is a trendy and nutritious breakfast option. Packed with healthy fats and protein, it's a satisfying meal that's easy to prepare.
Total Prep Time: 10 minutes

Ingredients:
- 1 slice whole-grain bread, toasted
- 1/2 ripe avocado, mashed
- 1 poached egg

- Salt and pepper to taste
- Red pepper flakes (optional)
- Fresh herbs for garnish (cilantro, chives)

Instructions:
1. Spread mashed avocado over the toasted bread.
2. Top with a poached egg.
3. Season with salt, pepper, and red pepper flakes if desired.
4. Garnish with fresh herbs.
5. Serve and enjoy.

Nutritional Information:
Calories: 280 | *Protein:* 13g | *Carbohydrates:* 20g | *Fat:* 18g | *Fiber:* 8g

Greek Yogurt Parfait with Walnuts and Honey

Intro: This Greek Yogurt Parfait is a delightful combination of creamy yogurt, crunchy walnuts, and sweet honey. It's a protein-packed breakfast that satisfies your sweet cravings.

Total Prep Time: 8 minutes

Ingredients:
- 1 cup Greek yogurt
- 1/4 cup chopped walnuts
- 1/2 cup mixed berries
- 1 tablespoon honey
- Granola (optional)

Instructions:

1. In a glass or bowl, layer Greek yogurt, walnuts, and berries.
2. Drizzle with honey.
3. Repeat the layers.
4. Top with granola if desired.
5. Serve chilled and enjoy.

Nutritional Information:

Calories: 320 | *Protein:* 20g | *Carbohydrates:* 25g | *Fat:* 15g | *Fiber:* 5g

Spinach and Mushroom Omelette

Intro: Start your day with a protein-packed Spinach and Mushroom Omelette. Loaded with veggies, it's a nutritious and flavorful breakfast that keeps you satisfied.

Total Prep Time: 15 minutes

Ingredients:

- 3 eggs
- 1/2 cup fresh spinach, chopped
- 1/4 cup mushrooms, sliced
- 1/4 cup feta cheese, crumbled
- Salt and pepper to taste
- Olive oil for cooking

Instructions:

1. Whisk eggs in a bowl and season with salt and pepper.
2. Heat olive oil in a pan over medium heat.
3. Add spinach and mushrooms, cook until wilted.
4. Pour whisked eggs over the veggies.
5. Sprinkle feta cheese on top.

6. Cook until eggs are set, then fold in half.
7. Slide onto a plate and serve.

Nutritional Information:

Calories: 280 | *Protein:* 18g | *Carbohydrates:* 5g | *Fat:* 22g | *Fiber:* 2g

Chia Seed Pudding with Mixed Berries

Intro: Chia Seed Pudding with Mixed Berries is a nutritious and delicious make-ahead breakfast. Packed with omega-3 fatty acids and antioxidants, it's a perfect option for a busy morning.

Total Prep Time: 4 hours (includes chilling time)

Ingredients:
- 3 tablespoons chia seeds
- 1 cup almond milk
- 1/2 teaspoon vanilla extract
- 1 tablespoon maple syrup
- Mixed berries for topping

Instructions:
1. In a bowl, mix chia seeds, almond milk, vanilla extract, and maple syrup.
2. Stir well and refrigerate for at least 4 hours or overnight.
3. Stir the pudding before serving.
4. Top with mixed berries.
5. Enjoy this delightful and healthy pudding.

Nutritional Information:

Calories: 180 | *Protein:* 5g | *Carbohydrates:* 20g | *Fat:* 9g | *Fiber:* 10g

Salmon and Avocado Breakfast Wrap

Intro: This Salmon and Avocado Breakfast Wrap is a tasty combination of omega-3-rich salmon, creamy avocado, and fresh veggies. It's a satisfying and nutritious way to start your day.
Total Prep Time: 15 minutes

Ingredients:
- 1 whole-grain wrap
- 4 ounces smoked salmon
- 1/2 avocado, sliced
- 1/4 cup cucumber, thinly sliced
- 2 tablespoons cream cheese
- Fresh dill for garnish
- Lemon wedge for serving

Instructions:
1. Spread cream cheese on the whole-grain wrap.
2. Layer with smoked salmon, avocado, and cucumber.
3. Garnish with fresh dill.
4. Roll up the wrap and slice in half.
5. Serve with a lemon wedge.

Nutritional Information:
Calories: 350 | *Protein:* 20g | *Carbohydrates:* 25g | *Fat:* 18g | *Fiber:* 8g

Sweet Potato Hash with Turkey Sausage

Intro: Sweet Potato Hash with Turkey Sausage is a flavorful and nutrient-packed breakfast option. Packed with lean protein and complex carbs, it's a filling choice that keeps you energized.

Total Prep Time: 25 minutes

Ingredients:
- 1 sweet potato, peeled and diced
- 1/2 pound turkey sausage, crumbled
- 1 bell pepper, diced
- 1 onion, diced
- 2 tablespoons olive oil
- Salt and pepper to taste
- Fresh parsley for garnish

Instructions:
1. Heat olive oil in a skillet over medium heat.
2. Add sweet potato, turkey sausage, bell pepper, and onion.
3. Cook until sweet potato is tender and sausage is browned.
4. Season with salt and pepper.
5. Garnish with fresh parsley.
6. Serve warm and enjoy.

Nutritional Information:
Calories: 320 | *Protein:* 15g | *Carbohydrates:* 30g | *Fat:* 16g | *Fiber:* 5g

Oatmeal with Flaxseeds and Blueberries

Intro: This Oatmeal with Flaxseeds and Blueberries is a classic and nutritious breakfast choice. Loaded with fiber and antioxidants, it's a comforting dish that promotes heart health.

Total Prep Time: 10 minutes

Ingredients:

- 1/2 cup rolled oats
- 1 cup milk (dairy or plant-based)
- 1 tablespoon flaxseeds
- 1/2 cup blueberries
- 1 tablespoon honey or maple syrup
- Chopped nuts for topping (optional)

Instructions:

1. In a saucepan, combine oats and milk. Cook over medium heat.
2. Stir in flaxseeds and blueberries.
3. Cook until oats are creamy and blueberries burst.
4. Sweeten with honey or maple syrup.
5. Top with chopped nuts if desired.
6. Serve warm and enjoy.

Nutritional Information:

Calories: 300 | *Protein:* 10g | *Carbohydrates:* 45g | *Fat:* 8g | *Fiber:* 7g

Green Tea Infused Quinoa Bowl

Intro: Elevate your breakfast with this Green Tea Infused Quinoa Bowl. Packed with antioxidants and protein, it's a unique and wholesome way to start your day on a healthy note.

Total Prep Time: 15 minutes

Ingredients:

- 1/2 cup quinoa, rinsed
- 1 cup green tea (brewed and cooled)
- 1/4 cup sliced almonds
- 1 tablespoon honey

- 1/2 cup mixed berries
- Greek yogurt for topping

Instructions:
1. Cook quinoa according to package instructions, using green tea instead of water.
2. Fluff quinoa with a fork and let it cool slightly.
3. Top with sliced almonds, honey, and mixed berries.
4. Add a dollop of Greek yogurt on top.
5. Serve and savor the unique flavors.

Nutritional Information:
Calories: 280 | *Protein:* 10g | *Carbohydrates:* 40g | *Fat:* 8g | *Fiber:* 6g

Almond Butter and Banana Smoothie Bowl

Intro: This Almond Butter and Banana Smoothie Bowl is a creamy and nutritious way to start your day. Packed with protein, healthy fats, and natural sweetness, it's a satisfying breakfast that will keep you fueled.
Total Prep Time: 10 minutes

Ingredients:
- 2 frozen bananas
- 1/2 cup almond milk
- 2 tablespoons almond butter
- 1 tablespoon chia seeds
- Toppings: Sliced bananas, granola, and a drizzle of honey

Instructions:
1. In a blender, combine frozen bananas, almond milk, almond butter, and chia seeds.

2. Blend until smooth and creamy.
3. Pour into a bowl and top with sliced bananas, granola, and a drizzle of honey.
4. Enjoy with a spoon!

Nutritional Information:

Calories: 380 | *Protein:* 10g | *Carbohydrates:* 45g | *Fat:* 18g | *Fiber:* 8g

Veggie and Egg Muffins

Intro: These Veggie and Egg Muffins are a convenient and protein-packed breakfast option. Loaded with colorful vegetables and eggs, they are perfect for a grab-and-go morning.

Total Prep Time: 25 minutes

Ingredients:
- 6 eggs
- 1/2 cup bell peppers, diced
- 1/2 cup cherry tomatoes, halved
- 1/4 cup spinach, chopped
- Salt and pepper to taste
- 1/4 cup feta cheese (optional)

Instructions:
1. Preheat the oven to 350°F (175°C) and grease a muffin tin.
2. In a bowl, whisk eggs and season with salt and pepper.
3. Stir in diced bell peppers, cherry tomatoes, and chopped spinach.
4. Pour the egg mixture into muffin cups.
5. Sprinkle with feta cheese if desired.

6. Bake for 15-20 minutes or until the eggs are set.
7. Allow to cool slightly before serving.

Nutritional Information:
Calories: 150 | *Protein:* 12g | *Carbohydrates:* 5g | *Fat:* 10g
| *Fiber:* 2g

Buckwheat Pancakes with Applesauce

Intro: Buckwheat Pancakes with Applesauce are a wholesome and gluten-free twist on traditional pancakes. These pancakes are light, fluffy, and served with a naturally sweetened applesauce for a delightful breakfast.
Total Prep Time: 20 minutes

Ingredients:
- 1 cup buckwheat flour
- 1 teaspoon baking powder
- 1/2 teaspoon cinnamon
- 1 cup almond milk
- 1 egg
- 2 tablespoons applesauce
- 1 tablespoon maple syrup

Instructions:
1. In a bowl, whisk together buckwheat flour, baking powder, and cinnamon.
2. Add almond milk, egg, applesauce, and maple syrup. Mix until well combined.
3. Heat a griddle or pan over medium heat and lightly grease.
4. Pour 1/4 cup of batter for each pancake onto the griddle.

5. Cook until bubbles form on the surface, then flip and cook until golden brown.
6. Serve with additional applesauce and enjoy.

Nutritional Information:

Calories: 220 | *Protein:* 8g | *Carbohydrates:* 35g | *Fat:* 6g | *Fiber:* 6g

Breakfast Burrito with Black Beans and Salsa

Intro: Spice up your morning with this flavorful Breakfast Burrito filled with black beans, salsa, and eggs. It's a protein-packed, satisfying option that will keep you energized.

Total Prep Time: 15 minutes

Ingredients:
- 1 whole-grain tortilla
- 1/2 cup black beans, cooked
- 2 eggs, scrambled
- 1/4 cup salsa
- 1/4 cup shredded cheese
- Fresh cilantro for garnish

Instructions:
1. Warm the tortilla in a dry skillet or microwave.
2. In the center of the tortilla, layer black beans, scrambled eggs, salsa, and shredded cheese.
3. Fold in the sides and roll up the burrito.
4. Place the burrito seam-side down in the skillet to seal.
5. Cook until the tortilla is lightly browned.
6. Garnish with fresh cilantro and serve.

Nutritional Information:
Calories: 380 | *Protein:* 20g | *Carbohydrates:* 35g | *Fat:* 18g | *Fiber:* 8g

Coconut and Pineapple Smoothie

Intro: Transport yourself to a tropical paradise with this Coconut and Pineapple Smoothie. Packed with the goodness of coconut and the sweetness of pineapple, it's a refreshing breakfast option.

Total Prep Time: 8 minutes

Ingredients:
- 1 cup coconut milk
- 1/2 cup pineapple chunks
- 1/2 banana
- 1/4 cup shredded coconut
- Ice cubes (optional)

Instructions:
1. In a blender, combine coconut milk, pineapple chunks, banana, and shredded coconut.
2. Blend until smooth.
3. Add ice cubes if desired and blend again.
4. Pour into a glass and enjoy the tropical flavors.

Nutritional Information:
Calories: 280 | *Protein:* 2g | *Carbohydrates:* 30g | *Fat:* 18g | *Fiber:* 5g

Spinach and Feta Breakfast Wrap

Intro: This Spinach and Feta Breakfast Wrap is a savory and satisfying morning meal. Filled with sautéed spinach, creamy feta, and eggs, it's a flavorful way to kickstart your day.

Total Prep Time: 15 minutes

Ingredients:
- 1 whole-grain wrap
- 1 cup fresh spinach
- 2 eggs, scrambled
- 2 tablespoons feta cheese, crumbled
- Salt and pepper to taste
- Olive oil for cooking

Instructions:
1. In a pan, sauté fresh spinach in olive oil until wilted.
2. Season with salt and pepper.
3. In the same pan, scramble eggs until cooked.
4. Place the scrambled eggs on the whole-grain wrap.
5. Top with sautéed spinach and crumbled feta.
6. Roll up the wrap and enjoy!

Nutritional Information:
Calories: 320 | *Protein:* 15g | *Carbohydrates:* 25g | *Fat:* 18g | *Fiber:* 5g

Turmeric and Ginger Infused Rice Porridge

Intro: Turmeric and Ginger Infused Rice Porridge is a comforting and anti-inflammatory breakfast option. With the warmth of turmeric and the zing of ginger, it's a nourishing way to start your day.

Total Prep Time: 30 minutes

Ingredients:
- 1/2 cup brown rice
- 2 cups milk (dairy or plant-based)
- 1 teaspoon turmeric powder
- 1/2 teaspoon ground ginger
- 1 tablespoon honey
- Toppings: Chopped nuts, sliced banana

Instructions:
1. Cook brown rice in milk according to package instructions.
2. Stir in turmeric powder, ground ginger, and honey.
3. Simmer until the porridge reaches your desired consistency.
4. Top with chopped nuts and sliced banana.
5. Serve warm and savor the comforting flavors.

Nutritional Information:
Calories: 280 | *Protein:* 8g | *Carbohydrates:* 45g | *Fat:* 7g | *Fiber:* 5g

Cottage Cheese with Fresh Fruit

Intro: Cottage Cheese with Fresh Fruit is a simple and protein-rich breakfast that combines the creaminess of cottage cheese with the sweetness of seasonal fruits. It's a light and refreshing option.

Total Prep Time: 5 minutes

Ingredients:
- 1/2 cup cottage cheese
- 1/2 cup fresh fruit (berries, kiwi, pineapple)
- 1 tablespoon honey
- Mint leaves for garnish

Instructions:
1. In a bowl, scoop cottage cheese.
2. Top with fresh fruit.
3. Drizzle with honey.
4. Garnish with mint leaves.
5. Serve chilled and enjoy this quick and nutritious breakfast.

Nutritional Information:
Calories: 220 | *Protein:* 15g | *Carbohydrates:* 25g | *Fat:* 8g | *Fiber:* 3g

Whole Grain Toast with Smoked Salmon

Intro: Elevate your breakfast with this Whole Grain Toast with Smoked Salmon. With the richness of smoked salmon and the wholesome goodness of whole grain bread, it's a delicious and nutritious choice.
Total Prep Time: 10 minutes

Ingredients:
- 2 slices whole grain bread, toasted
- 2 ounces smoked salmon
- 2 tablespoons cream cheese
- Capers and fresh dill for garnish

Instructions:
1. Spread cream cheese on toasted whole grain bread slices.
2. Layer with smoked salmon.
3. Garnish with capers and fresh dill.
4. Serve open-faced and enjoy the indulgent flavors.

Nutritional Information:
Calories: 280 | *Protein:* 18g | *Carbohydrates:* 20g | *Fat:* 14g | *Fiber:* 4g

Blueberry and Walnut Muffins

Intro: These Blueberry and Walnut Muffins are a delightful combination of juicy blueberries and crunchy walnuts. Made with wholesome ingredients, they are a perfect grab-and-go breakfast or snack.
Total Prep Time: 30 minutes

Ingredients:
- 1 1/2 cups whole wheat flour
- 1/2 cup oats
- 1 teaspoon baking powder
- 1/2 teaspoon baking soda
- 1/4 teaspoon salt
- 1/2 cup unsweetened applesauce
- 1/4 cup melted coconut oil
- 1/4 cup maple syrup
- 2 eggs
- 1 cup blueberries
- 1/2 cup chopped walnuts

Instructions:
1. Preheat the oven to 350°F (175°C) and line a muffin tin with paper liners.
2. In a bowl, combine whole wheat flour, oats, baking powder, baking soda, and salt.
3. In another bowl, whisk together applesauce, melted coconut oil, maple syrup, and eggs.
4. Add the wet ingredients to the dry ingredients and mix until just combined.

5. Fold in blueberries and chopped walnuts.
6. Divide the batter among the muffin cups.
7. Bake for 20-25 minutes or until a toothpick inserted comes out clean.
8. Allow to cool before enjoying.

Nutritional Information:
Calories: 180 | *Protein:* 5g | *Carbohydrates:* 25g | *Fat:* 8g | *Fiber:* 3g

Mango and Kiwi Breakfast Salad

Intro: Start your day with a burst of tropical flavors with this Mango and Kiwi Breakfast Salad. Packed with vitamins and antioxidants, it's a refreshing and healthy way to enjoy a morning salad.

Total Prep Time: 10 minutes

Ingredients:
- 1 mango, peeled and diced
- 2 kiwis, peeled and sliced
- 1/2 cup Greek yogurt
- 2 tablespoons honey
- 2 tablespoons chopped mint

Instructions:
1. In a bowl, combine diced mango and sliced kiwi.
2. In a separate bowl, mix Greek yogurt and honey.
3. Pour the yogurt mixture over the fruit.
4. Sprinkle with chopped mint.
5. Gently toss to combine.
6. Serve chilled and savor the vibrant flavors.

Nutritional Information:
Calories: 220 | *Protein:* 6g | *Carbohydrates:* 45g | *Fat:* 2g
| *Fiber:* 6g

Sweet Potato and Kale Breakfast Skillet

Intro: This Sweet Potato and Kale Breakfast Skillet is a hearty and nutritious one-pan breakfast. Packed with sweet potatoes, kale, and eggs, it's a flavorful way to start your day.

Total Prep Time: 25 minutes

Ingredients:
- 1 sweet potato, peeled and diced
- 1 cup kale, chopped
- 1/2 onion, diced
- 2 eggs
- 1 tablespoon olive oil
- Salt and pepper to taste
- Hot sauce for garnish (optional)

Instructions:
1. In a skillet, heat olive oil over medium heat.
2. Add diced sweet potatoes and cook until slightly softened.
3. Add chopped kale and diced onion. Cook until vegetables are tender.
4. Create two wells in the mixture and crack eggs into each well.
5. Cover and cook until eggs are done to your liking.
6. Season with salt and pepper.
7. Garnish with hot sauce if desired.
8. Serve warm and enjoy this wholesome skillet.

Nutritional Information:

Calories: 320 | *Protein:* 12g | *Carbohydrates:* 35g | *Fat:* 16g | *Fiber:* 7g

Protein-Packed Lentil Breakfast Bowl

Intro: This Protein-Packed Lentil Breakfast Bowl is a savory and filling breakfast option. Loaded with protein and fiber from lentils, it's a nutritious way to fuel your day.
Total Prep Time: 20 minutes

Ingredients:
- 1/2 cup cooked lentils
- 1/4 cup cherry tomatoes, halved
- 1/4 cup cucumber, diced
- 1/4 cup feta cheese, crumbled
- 2 tablespoons balsamic vinaigrette
- Poached egg for topping (optional)

Instructions:
1. In a bowl, combine cooked lentils, cherry tomatoes, cucumber, and crumbled feta.
2. Drizzle with balsamic vinaigrette and toss to combine.
3. Top with a poached egg if desired.
4. Serve and enjoy this protein-packed breakfast bowl.

Nutritional Information:

Calories: 300 | *Protein:* 18g | *Carbohydrates:* 30g | *Fat:* 12g | *Fiber:* 8g

Pumpkin Seed Granola with Yogurt

Intro: Pumpkin Seed Granola with Yogurt is a crunchy and nutrient-rich breakfast option. Packed with the goodness of oats, seeds, and yogurt, it's a delightful way to add texture and flavor to your morning routine.
Total Prep Time: 25 minutes

Ingredients:
- 2 cups old-fashioned oats
- 1/2 cup pumpkin seeds
- 1/4 cup honey
- 2 tablespoons coconut oil, melted
- 1 teaspoon vanilla extract
- Pinch of salt
- Greek yogurt for serving
- Fresh berries for topping

Instructions:
1. Preheat the oven to 325°F (163°C) and line a baking sheet with parchment paper.
2. In a bowl, mix oats, pumpkin seeds, honey, melted coconut oil, vanilla extract, and a pinch of salt.
3. Spread the mixture evenly on the prepared baking sheet.
4. Bake for 20-25 minutes, stirring halfway through, until golden brown.
5. Allow the granola to cool completely.
6. Serve with Greek yogurt and top with fresh berries.

Nutritional Information:
Calories: 280 | *Protein:* 8g | *Carbohydrates:* 35g | *Fat:* 12g | *Fiber:* 6g

Broccoli and Cheese Breakfast Casserole

Intro: This Broccoli and Cheese Breakfast Casserole is a wholesome and satisfying way to start your day. Packed with protein, veggies, and cheesy goodness, it's a crowd-pleaser for breakfast or brunch.

Total Prep Time: 45 minutes

Ingredients:
- 2 cups broccoli florets, steamed
- 1 cup cooked quinoa
- 6 eggs
- 1 cup milk (dairy or plant-based)
- 1 1/2 cups shredded cheddar cheese
- Salt and pepper to taste
- 1/4 teaspoon garlic powder
- 1/4 teaspoon onion powder

Instructions:
1. Preheat the oven to 375°F (190°C) and grease a baking dish.
2. In a bowl, whisk together eggs, milk, salt, pepper, garlic powder, and onion powder.
3. Spread cooked quinoa in the bottom of the baking dish.
4. Arrange steamed broccoli over the quinoa.
5. Pour the egg mixture over the broccoli and quinoa.
6. Sprinkle shredded cheddar cheese on top.
7. Bake for 30-35 minutes or until the center is set and the top is golden.
8. Allow the casserole to cool slightly before slicing and serving.

Nutritional Information:
Calories: 320 | *Protein:* 18g | *Carbohydrates:* 20g | *Fat:* 18g | *Fiber:* 3g

Grilled Chicken Salad with Mixed Greens

Intro: Indulge in the freshness of a Grilled Chicken Salad with Mixed Greens. This vibrant salad combines the juiciness of grilled chicken with a medley of mixed greens, creating a wholesome and satisfying meal.
Total Prep Time: 30 minutes

Ingredients:
- 1 pound boneless, skinless chicken breasts
- 6 cups mixed salad greens
- Cherry tomatoes, halved
- Cucumber, sliced
- Red onion, thinly sliced
- Balsamic vinaigrette dressing
- Salt and pepper to taste

Instructions:
1. Season chicken breasts with salt and pepper.
2. Grill the chicken until fully cooked, then slice.
3. In a large bowl, combine mixed salad greens, cherry tomatoes, cucumber, and red onion.
4. Top with grilled chicken slices.
5. Drizzle with balsamic vinaigrette dressing.
6. Toss gently to combine.
7. Serve immediately and enjoy this refreshing salad.

Nutritional Information:
Calories: 350 | *Protein:* 30g | *Carbohydrates:* 15g | *Fat:* 18g | *Fiber:* 5g

Lentil and Vegetable Soup

Intro: Embrace comfort with a hearty Lentil and Vegetable Soup. This wholesome soup is a medley of lentils and vibrant vegetables, simmered to perfection, creating a nourishing bowl of goodness.
Total Prep Time: 40 minutes

Ingredients:
- 1 cup dried lentils, rinsed
- 1 onion, diced
- 2 carrots, chopped
- 2 celery stalks, chopped
- 3 cloves garlic, minced
- 6 cups vegetable broth
- 1 can (14 oz) diced tomatoes
- 1 teaspoon ground cumin
- 1 teaspoon smoked paprika
- Salt and pepper to taste
- Fresh parsley for garnish

Instructions:
1. In a large pot, sauté onion, carrots, celery, and garlic until softened.
2. Add lentils, vegetable broth, diced tomatoes, cumin, smoked paprika, salt, and pepper.
3. Bring to a boil, then reduce heat and simmer for 30 minutes or until lentils are tender.
4. Adjust seasoning if needed.
5. Garnish with fresh parsley.
6. Serve hot and savor the comforting flavors.

Nutritional Information:
Calories: 250 | *Protein:* 15g | *Carbohydrates:* 40g | *Fat:* 2g | *Fiber:* 15g

Quinoa and Black Bean Stuffed Peppers

Intro: Elevate your meal with Quinoa and Black Bean Stuffed Peppers. These colorful peppers are filled with a wholesome mix of quinoa, black beans, and flavorful spices, creating a delicious and nutritious dish.
Total Prep Time: 45 minutes

Ingredients:
- 4 bell peppers, halved and seeds removed
- 1 cup quinoa, cooked
- 1 can (15 oz) black beans, drained and rinsed
- 1 cup corn kernels (fresh or frozen)
- 1 cup diced tomatoes
- 1 teaspoon cumin
- 1 teaspoon chili powder
- Salt and pepper to taste
- Shredded cheese for topping
- Fresh cilantro for garnish

Instructions:
1. Preheat the oven to 375°F (190°C).
2. In a bowl, mix cooked quinoa, black beans, corn, diced tomatoes, cumin, chili powder, salt, and pepper.
3. Stuff each bell pepper half with the quinoa and black bean mixture.
4. Top with shredded cheese.
5. Bake for 25-30 minutes or until peppers are tender and cheese is melted.

6. Garnish with fresh cilantro.
7. Serve and enjoy this flavorful stuffed peppers dish.

Nutritional Information:
Calories: 320 | *Protein:* 15g | *Carbohydrates:* 55g | *Fat:* 5g | *Fiber:* 12g

Salmon and Avocado Salad

Intro: Delight your taste buds with a Salmon and Avocado Salad. This refreshing salad combines flaky salmon, creamy avocado, and crisp greens, creating a nutritious and satisfying meal.

Total Prep Time: 20 minutes

Ingredients:
- 8 oz salmon fillet, grilled or baked
- 4 cups mixed salad greens
- 1 avocado, sliced
- Cherry tomatoes, halved
- Cucumber, sliced
- Lemon vinaigrette dressing
- Salt and pepper to taste

Instructions:
1. Grill or bake the salmon until fully cooked.
2. In a large bowl, combine mixed salad greens, avocado slices, cherry tomatoes, and cucumber.
3. Flake the cooked salmon and add it to the salad.
4. Drizzle with lemon vinaigrette dressing.
5. Season with salt and pepper to taste.
6. Toss gently to combine.
7. Serve immediately and enjoy this light and flavorful salad.

Spinach and Chickpea Wrap

Intro: Savor the goodness of a Spinach and Chickpea Wrap. Filled with nutrient-packed spinach, protein-rich chickpeas, and a flavorful tahini dressing, it's a wholesome and satisfying wrap for any meal.
Total Prep Time: 15 minutes

Ingredients:
- 1 whole-grain wrap
- 1 cup fresh spinach leaves
- 1/2 cup chickpeas, cooked
- 1/4 cup cherry tomatoes, halved
- Red onion, thinly sliced
- Feta cheese, crumbled
- Tahini dressing
- Salt and pepper to taste

Instructions:
1. Lay the whole-grain wrap on a flat surface.
2. Arrange fresh spinach leaves, chickpeas, cherry tomatoes, red onion, and crumbled feta on the wrap.
3. Drizzle with tahini dressing.
4. Season with salt and pepper to taste.
5. Fold in the sides and roll up the wrap.
6. Slice in half and serve this nutritious and flavorful wrap.

Nutritional Information:
Calories: 320 | *Protein:* 12g | *Carbohydrates:* 45g | *Fat:* 12g | *Fiber:* 8g

Turkey and Vegetable Stir-Fry

Intro: Enjoy a quick and nutritious Turkey and Vegetable Stir-Fry. This flavorful stir-fry combines lean turkey with colorful vegetables, creating a protein-packed meal that's perfect for busy days.

Total Prep Time: 25 minutes

Ingredients:
- 1 pound ground turkey
- 2 cups broccoli florets
- 1 bell pepper, thinly sliced
- 1 carrot, julienned
- 2 cloves garlic, minced
- 1/4 cup soy sauce
- 1 tablespoon sesame oil
- 1 tablespoon hoisin sauce
- Green onions for garnish
- Sesame seeds for garnish

Instructions:
1. In a wok or large skillet, cook ground turkey until browned.
2. Add broccoli, bell pepper, carrot, and minced garlic to the skillet.
3. In a small bowl, mix soy sauce, sesame oil, and hoisin sauce.
4. Pour the sauce over the turkey and vegetables.
5. Stir-fry until the vegetables are tender and the sauce coats everything.

6. Garnish with chopped green onions and sesame seeds.
7. Serve over rice or quinoa and enjoy this quick and delicious stir-fry.

Nutritional Information:
Calories: 350 | *Protein:* 25g | *Carbohydrates:* 20g | *Fat:* 18g | *Fiber:* 6g

Sweet Potato and Lentil Curry

Intro: Warm your soul with a Sweet Potato and Lentil Curry. This aromatic and hearty curry combines sweet potatoes, lentils, and a blend of spices, creating a comforting and nutritious dish.
Total Prep Time: 40 minutes

Ingredients:
- 1 cup dried lentils, rinsed
- 2 sweet potatoes, peeled and diced
- 1 onion, finely chopped
- 3 cloves garlic, minced
- 1 can (14 oz) diced tomatoes
- 1 can (14 oz) coconut milk
- 2 tablespoons curry powder
- 1 teaspoon ground turmeric
- 1 teaspoon cumin
- Salt and pepper to taste
- Fresh cilantro for garnish
- Cooked rice for serving

Instructions:
1. In a large pot, sauté chopped onion and minced garlic until softened.

2. Add diced sweet potatoes, dried lentils, diced tomatoes, coconut milk, curry powder, turmeric, cumin, salt, and pepper.
3. Bring to a boil, then reduce heat and simmer until lentils and sweet potatoes are tender.
4. Adjust seasoning if needed.
5. Serve over cooked rice.
6. Garnish with fresh cilantro.
7. Enjoy this flavorful and comforting curry.

Nutritional Information:
Calories: 380 | *Protein:* 15g | *Carbohydrates:* 55g | *Fat:* 12g | *Fiber:* 12g

Mediterranean Quinoa Salad

Intro: Transport your taste buds to the Mediterranean with a refreshing Quinoa Salad. Packed with quinoa, colorful vegetables, olives, and feta cheese, it's a light and flavorful dish that's perfect for any occasion.
Total Prep Time: 25 minutes

Ingredients:
- 1 cup quinoa, cooked
- 1 cucumber, diced
- Cherry tomatoes, halved
- Kalamata olives, sliced
- Red onion, finely chopped
- Feta cheese, crumbled
- Fresh parsley, chopped
- Lemon vinaigrette dressing
- Salt and pepper to taste

Instructions:

1. In a large bowl, combine cooked quinoa, diced cucumber, cherry tomatoes, olives, red onion, and crumbled feta.
2. Drizzle with lemon vinaigrette dressing.
3. Season with salt and pepper to taste.
4. Toss gently to combine.
5. Garnish with fresh parsley.
6. Serve chilled and enjoy this Mediterranean-inspired quinoa salad.

Nutritional Information:
Calories: 320 | *Protein:* 10g | *Carbohydrates:* 45g | *Fat:* 12g | *Fiber:* 8g

Chicken and Vegetable Quinoa Bowl

Intro: Create a balanced and satisfying meal with a Chicken and Vegetable Quinoa Bowl. Loaded with grilled chicken, roasted vegetables, and fluffy quinoa, it's a wholesome bowl that will leave you feeling nourished.
Total Prep Time: 30 minutes

Ingredients:

- 1 cup quinoa, cooked
- 1 pound boneless, skinless chicken breasts, grilled
- 2 cups mixed vegetables (bell peppers, zucchini, cherry tomatoes), roasted
- 1 avocado, sliced
- Olive oil for drizzling
- Balsamic glaze for topping
- Salt and pepper to taste

Instructions:

1. Cook quinoa according to package instructions.
2. Grill chicken until fully cooked, then slice.
3. Roast mixed vegetables in the oven until tender.
4. In a bowl, assemble quinoa, grilled chicken, roasted vegetables, and sliced avocado.
5. Drizzle with olive oil and balsamic glaze.
6. Season with salt and pepper to taste.
7. Toss gently to combine.
8. Serve this hearty quinoa bowl and enjoy a balanced and delicious meal.

Nutritional Information:

Calories: 380 | *Protein:* 30g | *Carbohydrates:* 35g | *Fat:* 15g | *Fiber:* 8g

Broccoli and Almond Soup

Intro: Warm up with a bowl of comforting Broccoli and Almond Soup. This velvety soup combines the goodness of broccoli with the richness of almonds, creating a nourishing and flavorful dish.

Total Prep Time: 35 minutes

Ingredients:

- 4 cups broccoli florets
- 1 onion, chopped
- 2 cloves garlic, minced
- 1/2 cup almonds, toasted
- 4 cups vegetable broth
- 1 cup almond milk
- Salt and pepper to taste
- Lemon zest for garnish

Instructions:
1. In a large pot, sauté chopped onion and minced garlic until softened.
2. Add broccoli florets, toasted almonds, vegetable broth, and almond milk.
3. Bring to a boil, then reduce heat and simmer until broccoli is tender.
4. Use an immersion blender to blend the soup until smooth.
5. Season with salt and pepper to taste.
6. Ladle the soup into bowls.
7. Garnish with lemon zest.
8. Serve hot and enjoy this creamy and nutty broccoli soup.

Nutritional Information:
Calories: 250 | *Protein:* 10g | *Carbohydrates:* 20g | *Fat:* 16g | *Fiber:* 8g

Shrimp and Avocado Lettuce Wraps

Intro: Delight your senses with Shrimp and Avocado Lettuce Wraps. These light and refreshing wraps combine succulent shrimp with creamy avocado, all nestled in crisp lettuce leaves for a perfect balance of flavors.
Total Prep Time: 20 minutes

Ingredients:
- 1 pound shrimp, cooked and peeled
- 2 avocados, sliced
- Bibb lettuce leaves
- Cherry tomatoes, halved
- Red onion, thinly sliced
- Cilantro for garnish

- Lime wedges
- Salt and pepper to taste

Instructions:
1. Arrange shrimp, avocado slices, cherry tomatoes, and red onion on lettuce leaves.
2. Squeeze lime wedges over the wraps.
3. Season with salt and pepper.
4. Garnish with cilantro.
5. Serve immediately and enjoy this light and flavorful dish.

Nutritional Information:
Calories: 280 | *Protein:* 25g | *Carbohydrates:* 12g | *Fat:* 16g | *Fiber:* 8g

Tofu and Vegetable Skewers

Intro: Elevate your grill game with Tofu and Vegetable Skewers. These skewers feature marinated tofu and a colorful mix of veggies, creating a delicious and plant-powered dish.

Total Prep Time: 30 minutes

Ingredients:
- 1 block extra-firm tofu, pressed and cubed
- Bell peppers, assorted colors, cut into chunks
- Zucchini, sliced
- Cherry tomatoes
- Red onion, cut into wedges
- Olive oil
- Soy sauce
- Garlic powder
- Smoked paprika

- Wooden skewers, soaked in water

Instructions:
1. In a bowl, mix olive oil, soy sauce, garlic powder, and smoked paprika.
2. Thread tofu and veggies onto the skewers.
3. Brush with the marinade.
4. Grill until tofu is golden and veggies are tender.
5. Serve these flavorful skewers as a delightful and wholesome meal.

Nutritional Information:
Calories: 220 | *Protein:* 15g | *Carbohydrates:* 20g | *Fat:* 12g | *Fiber:* 8g

Kale and White Bean Salad

Intro: Nourish your body with a Kale and White Bean Salad. Packed with nutrient-rich kale, protein-packed white beans, and a zesty dressing, it's a hearty and satisfying salad.

Total Prep Time: 15 minutes

Ingredients:
- 4 cups kale, chopped
- 1 can (15 oz) white beans, drained and rinsed
- Cherry tomatoes, halved
- Red bell pepper, diced
- Feta cheese, crumbled
- Kalamata olives, sliced
- Olive oil
- Lemon juice
- Dijon mustard
- Garlic, minced

- Salt and pepper to taste

Instructions:
1. In a large bowl, combine chopped kale, white beans, cherry tomatoes, red bell pepper, feta cheese, and olives.
2. In a small bowl, whisk together olive oil, lemon juice, Dijon mustard, minced garlic, salt, and pepper.
3. Pour the dressing over the salad and toss to combine.
4. Serve this nutritious and flavorful Kale and White Bean Salad.

Nutritional Information:
Calories: 280 | *Protein:* 15g | *Carbohydrates:* 30g | *Fat:* 12g | *Fiber:* 10g

Lemon Garlic Grilled Salmon

Intro: Enjoy the simplicity and elegance of Lemon Garlic Grilled Salmon. This classic dish features succulent salmon fillets marinated in a zesty lemon and garlic mixture, grilled to perfection for a delightful and healthy meal.
Total Prep Time: 25 minutes

Ingredients:
- 4 salmon fillets
- Lemon zest
- Lemon juice
- Garlic, minced
- Olive oil
- Fresh dill, chopped
- Salt and pepper to taste

Instructions:
1. In a bowl, mix lemon zest, lemon juice, minced garlic, olive oil, chopped fresh dill, salt, and pepper.
2. Coat salmon fillets with the marinade.
3. Grill until salmon is cooked to your liking.
4. Garnish with additional dill and lemon slices.
5. Serve this Lemon Garlic Grilled Salmon for a light and flavorful meal.

Nutritional Information:
Calories: 320 | *Protein:* 30g | *Carbohydrates:* 2g | *Fat:* 22g | *Fiber:* 0g

Cauliflower and Chickpea Curry

Intro: Dive into the rich and aromatic flavors of Cauliflower and Chickpea Curry. This vegetarian dish combines tender cauliflower, hearty chickpeas, and a flavorful curry sauce for a comforting and satisfying meal.
Total Prep Time: 40 minutes

Ingredients:
- 1 cauliflower, cut into florets
- 1 can (15 oz) chickpeas, drained and rinsed
- Onion, finely chopped
- Garlic, minced
- Ginger, grated
- Tomato puree
- Coconut milk
- Curry powder
- Turmeric
- Cumin
- Coriander
- Cayenne pepper (optional)

- Fresh cilantro for garnish
- Cooked rice for serving

Instructions:

1. In a pan, sauté chopped onion, minced garlic, and grated ginger until fragrant.
2. Add curry powder, turmeric, cumin, coriander, and cayenne pepper. Cook for a minute.
3. Stir in cauliflower florets and chickpeas.
4. Add tomato puree and coconut milk. Simmer until cauliflower is tender.
5. Adjust seasoning if needed.
6. Garnish with fresh cilantro.
7. Serve this Cauliflower and Chickpea Curry over rice for a flavorful experience.

Nutritional Information:

Calories: 300 | *Protein:* 12g | *Carbohydrates:* 40g | *Fat:* 10g | *Fiber:* 10g

Turkey and Quinoa Stuffed Bell Peppers

Intro: Enjoy a wholesome and satisfying meal with Turkey and Quinoa Stuffed Bell Peppers. These vibrant peppers are filled with a flavorful mix of lean ground turkey, quinoa, and a medley of vegetables.

Total Prep Time: 50 minutes

Ingredients:

- 4 bell peppers, halved and seeds removed
- 1 cup quinoa, cooked
- 1 pound lean ground turkey
- Onion, finely chopped
- Garlic, minced

- Diced tomatoes
- Black beans, drained and rinsed
- Corn kernels (fresh or frozen)
- Taco seasoning
- Shredded cheese for topping
- Fresh cilantro for garnish

Instructions:
1. Preheat the oven to 375°F (190°C).
2. In a skillet, cook ground turkey until browned.
3. Add chopped onion and minced garlic. Cook until softened.
4. Stir in cooked quinoa, diced tomatoes, black beans, corn, and taco seasoning.
5. Fill each bell pepper half with the turkey and quinoa mixture.
6. Top with shredded cheese.
7. Bake for 25-30 minutes or until peppers are tender and cheese is melted.
8. Garnish with fresh cilantro.
9. Serve these Turkey and Quinoa Stuffed Bell Peppers for a nutritious and flavorful dinner.

Nutritional Information:
Calories: 350 | *Protein:* 25g | *Carbohydrates:* 35g | *Fat:* 12g | *Fiber:* 8g

Greek Chicken Souvlaki Bowl

Intro: Transport your taste buds to the Mediterranean with a Greek Chicken Souvlaki Bowl. This bowl features marinated chicken, quinoa, and a medley of fresh vegetables, all topped with a tangy tzatziki sauce for a delightful and healthy meal.

Total Prep Time: 35 minutes

Ingredients:
- 1 pound chicken breasts, cubed
- Greek yogurt
- Lemon juice
- Garlic, minced
- Oregano
- Cucumber, diced
- Cherry tomatoes, halved
- Red onion, thinly sliced
- Kalamata olives, sliced
- Feta cheese, crumbled
- Quinoa, cooked
- Tzatziki sauce for topping

Instructions:
1. In a bowl, mix Greek yogurt, lemon juice, minced garlic, and oregano.
2. Marinate chicken cubes in the mixture for at least 30 minutes.
3. Grill the chicken until fully cooked.
4. In a bowl, assemble cooked quinoa, grilled chicken, cucumber, cherry tomatoes, red onion, olives, and crumbled feta.
5. Drizzle with tzatziki sauce.
6. Toss gently to combine.
7. Serve this Greek Chicken Souvlaki Bowl for a taste of the Mediterranean.

Nutritional Information:
Calories: 380 | *Protein:* 30g | *Carbohydrates:* 30g | *Fat:* 15g | *Fiber:* 6g

Spaghetti Squash with Tomato Basil Sauce

Intro: Swap traditional pasta for Spaghetti Squash with Tomato Basil Sauce. This low-carb and nutritious dish feature strands of roasted spaghetti squash topped with a vibrant and herb-infused tomato basil sauce.
Total Prep Time: 50 minutes

Ingredients:
- 1 spaghetti squash, halved and seeds removed
- Olive oil
- Salt and pepper to taste
- 2 cups tomato sauce
- Fresh basil, chopped
- Garlic, minced
- Red pepper flakes (optional)
- Grated Parmesan cheese for topping

Instructions:
1. Preheat the oven to 400°F (200°C).
2. Drizzle spaghetti squash halves with olive oil and season with salt and pepper.
3. Roast for 40-45 minutes or until the squash is fork-tender.
4. Meanwhile, in a saucepan, heat tomato sauce, chopped basil, minced garlic, and red pepper flakes if desired.
5. Scrape the spaghetti squash with a fork to create strands.
6. Serve the spaghetti squash topped with tomato basil sauce.
7. Sprinkle with grated Parmesan cheese.
8. Enjoy this wholesome and satisfying Spaghetti Squash with Tomato Basil Sauce.

Nutritional Information:
Calories: 220 | *Protein:* 6g | *Carbohydrates:* 40g | *Fat:* 8g | *Fiber:* 10g

Avocado and Black Bean Salad

Intro: Refresh your palate with Avocado and Black Bean Salad. This vibrant and nutrient-packed salad combines creamy avocado, black beans, corn, and a zesty lime dressing for a light and flavorful dish.

Total Prep Time: 20 minutes

Ingredients:

- 2 avocados, diced
- 1 can (15 oz) black beans, drained and rinsed
- Corn kernels (fresh or frozen)
- Red onion, finely chopped
- Cherry tomatoes, halved
- Fresh cilantro, chopped
- Lime juice
- Olive oil
- Salt and pepper to taste

Instructions:

1. In a bowl, combine diced avocado, black beans, corn, chopped red onion, cherry tomatoes, and cilantro.
2. In a small bowl, whisk together lime juice, olive oil, salt, and pepper.
3. Drizzle the dressing over the salad and toss gently to combine.
4. Serve this Avocado and Black Bean Salad as a refreshing side or a light meal.

Nutritional Information:
Calories: 280 | *Protein:* 10g | *Carbohydrates:* 35g | *Fat:* 14g | *Fiber:* 12g

Asparagus and Mushroom Quiche

Intro: Embrace brunch with the delightful Asparagus and Mushroom Quiche. This savory and cheesy quiche features a flaky crust filled with tender asparagus, mushrooms, and a rich egg custard for a satisfying meal.
Total Prep Time: 1 hour

Ingredients:
- 1 pre-made pie crust
- Asparagus spears, trimmed
- Mushrooms, sliced
- Onion, finely chopped
- 6 eggs
- Milk
- Shredded Swiss cheese
- Salt and pepper to taste
- Fresh chives for garnish

Instructions:
1. Preheat the oven to 375°F (190°C).
2. Roll out the pie crust and press it into a quiche dish.
3. In a skillet, sauté chopped onion, mushrooms, and asparagus until tender.
4. In a bowl, whisk together eggs, milk, shredded Swiss cheese, salt, and pepper.
5. Arrange the sautéed vegetables in the pie crust.
6. Pour the egg mixture over the vegetables.
7. Bake for 35-40 minutes or until the quiche is set and golden.

8. Garnish with fresh chives.
9. Allow to cool slightly before slicing and serving this Asparagus and Mushroom Quiche.

Nutritional Information:
Calories: 320 | *Protein:* 15g | *Carbohydrates:* 20g | *Fat:* 18g | *Fiber:* 3g

Turkey and Sweet Potato Chili

Intro: Warm up with a bowl of comforting Turkey and Sweet Potato Chili. This hearty and nutritious chili features lean ground turkey, sweet potatoes, beans, and a medley of spices for a flavorful and satisfying meal.
Total Prep Time: 45 minutes

Ingredients:
- 1 pound lean ground turkey
- Sweet potatoes, peeled and diced
- Onion, finely chopped
- Garlic, minced
- Black beans, drained and rinsed
- Kidney beans, drained and rinsed
- Diced tomatoes
- Tomato paste
- Chili powder
- Cumin
- Paprika
- Cayenne pepper (optional)
- Salt and pepper to taste
- Greek yogurt for topping
- Fresh cilantro for garnish

Instructions:

1. In a large pot, cook ground turkey until browned.
2. Add chopped onion and minced garlic. Cook until softened.
3. Stir in diced sweet potatoes, black beans, kidney beans, diced tomatoes, tomato paste, chili powder, cumin, paprika, cayenne pepper, salt, and pepper.
4. Simmer until sweet potatoes are tender and the flavors meld, approximately 30 minutes.
5. Adjust seasoning if needed.
6. Serve the Turkey and Sweet Potato Chili hot, topped with a dollop of Greek yogurt and garnished with fresh cilantro.
7. Enjoy the heartiness and warmth of this comforting chili.

Nutritional Information:

Calories: 350 | *Protein:* 25g | *Carbohydrates:* 40g | *Fat:* 10g | *Fiber:* 12g

Brown Rice Bowl with Tuna and Avocado

Intro: Create a balanced and satisfying Brown Rice Bowl with Tuna and Avocado. This wholesome bowl features nutrient-rich brown rice, flaky tuna, creamy avocado, and a drizzle of soy-ginger dressing for a delicious and nutritious meal.

Total Prep Time: 25 minutes

Ingredients:

- 2 cups brown rice, cooked
- Canned tuna, drained
- Avocado, sliced
- Cucumber, julienned

- Carrot, shredded
- Edamame, steamed
- Soy-ginger dressing
- Sesame seeds for topping
- Nori strips for garnish

Instructions:
1. In a bowl, assemble cooked brown rice, canned tuna, avocado slices, julienned cucumber, shredded carrot, and steamed edamame.
2. Drizzle with soy-ginger dressing.
3. Sprinkle sesame seeds over the bowl.
4. Garnish with nori strips.
5. Toss gently to combine.
6. Serve this Brown Rice Bowl with Tuna and Avocado for a well-rounded and flavorful dish.

Nutritional Information:
Calories: 380 | *Protein:* 20g | *Carbohydrates:* 50g | *Fat:* 15g | *Fiber:* 8g

Eggplant and Tomato Stack

Intro: Elevate your vegetable game with the Eggplant and Tomato Stack. This elegant dish features layers of grilled eggplant, ripe tomatoes, and melted mozzarella, drizzled with balsamic glaze for a delightful and visually appealing meal.

Total Prep Time: 30 minutes

Ingredients:
- Eggplant, sliced
- Ripe tomatoes, sliced
- Fresh mozzarella, sliced

- Balsamic glaze
- Fresh basil leaves
- Olive oil
- Salt and pepper to taste

Instructions:
1. Preheat a grill or grill pan.
2. Brush eggplant slices with olive oil and season with salt and pepper.
3. Grill the eggplant until tender and grill marks appear.
4. Assemble stacks by layering grilled eggplant, sliced tomatoes, and fresh mozzarella.
5. Drizzle with balsamic glaze.
6. Garnish with fresh basil leaves.
7. Serve the Eggplant and Tomato Stack as a flavorful and elegant side or appetizer.

Nutritional Information:
Calories: 250 | *Protein:* 12g | *Carbohydrates:* 20g | *Fat:* 15g | *Fiber:* 8g

Pesto Zucchini Noodles with Cherry Tomatoes

Intro: Embrace a low-carb delight with Pesto Zucchini Noodles with Cherry Tomatoes. These zucchini noodles, or "zoodles," are tossed in a vibrant pesto sauce and paired with juicy cherry tomatoes for a light and flavorful dish.
Total Prep Time: 15 minutes

Ingredients:
- Zucchini, spiralized into noodles
- Cherry tomatoes, halved

- Pesto sauce
- Pine nuts for topping
- Parmesan cheese for garnish
- Fresh basil leaves for garnish
- Salt and pepper to taste

Instructions:
1. Spiralize zucchini into noodles.
2. In a bowl, toss zucchini noodles with cherry tomatoes and pesto sauce.
3. Season with salt and pepper to taste.
4. Top with pine nuts, Parmesan cheese, and fresh basil leaves.
5. Serve these Pesto Zucchini Noodles for a light and satisfying meal.

Nutritional Information:
Calories: 220 | *Protein:* 8g | *Carbohydrates:* 15g | *Fat:* 18g | *Fiber:* 5g

Chickpea and Spinach Quesadilla

Intro: Spice up your meal with a Chickpea and Spinach Quesadilla. This flavorful quesadilla combines protein-packed chickpeas, sautéed spinach, and melted cheese for a quick and satisfying dish.
Total Prep Time: 20 minutes

Ingredients:
- Flour tortillas
- Chickpeas, cooked
- Fresh spinach leaves
- Shredded cheese (cheddar or Mexican blend)
- Olive oil

- Cumin
- Paprika
- Garlic powder
- Salt and pepper to taste
- Salsa and Greek yogurt for dipping

Instructions:
1. In a skillet, sauté chickpeas in olive oil with cumin, paprika, garlic powder, salt, and pepper until heated through.
2. Remove chickpeas from the skillet and set aside.
3. In the same skillet, wilt fresh spinach leaves.
4. On a tortilla, layer shredded cheese, sautéed spinach, and chickpeas.
5. Top with another tortilla.
6. Cook on both sides until the tortilla is golden and the cheese is melted.
7. Slice and serve with salsa and Greek yogurt for dipping.
8. Enjoy this Chickpea and Spinach Quesadilla as a flavorful and satisfying meal.

Nutritional Information:
Calories: 320 | *Protein:* 15g | *Carbohydrates:* 35g | *Fat:* 15g | *Fiber:* 8g

Baked Cod with Lemon and Dill

Intro: Savor the flavors of the sea with Baked Cod with Lemon and Dill. This simple and wholesome dish features cod fillets seasoned with zesty lemon and aromatic dill, baked to perfection for a light and nutritious meal.
Total Prep Time: 25 minutes

Ingredients:

- Cod fillets
- Lemon, sliced
- Fresh dill, chopped
- Olive oil
- Garlic powder
- Salt and pepper to taste

Instructions:

1. Preheat the oven to 375°F (190°C).
2. Place cod fillets on a baking sheet.
3. Drizzle with olive oil and sprinkle with garlic powder, salt, and pepper.
4. Arrange lemon slices on top of the fillets.
5. Bake for 15-20 minutes or until the cod is cooked through.
6. Garnish with chopped fresh dill.
7. Serve this Baked Cod with Lemon and Dill with your favorite side dishes.

Nutritional Information:

Calories: 220 | *Protein:* 25g | *Carbohydrates:* 2g | *Fat:* 12g | *Fiber:* 1g

Quinoa and Vegetable Stir-Fry

Intro: Stir up a rainbow of colors and flavors with Quinoa and Vegetable Stir-Fry. This vibrant and nutrient-packed dish combines fluffy quinoa with a medley of fresh vegetables, stir-fried to perfection and seasoned with a savory sauce.

Total Prep Time: 30 minutes

Ingredients:
- 1 cup quinoa, cooked
- Mixed vegetables (broccoli, bell peppers, carrots, snap peas), chopped
- Soy sauce
- Sesame oil
- Garlic, minced
- Ginger, grated
- Green onions, sliced
- Sesame seeds for topping

Instructions:
1. In a wok or large skillet, heat sesame oil.
2. Sauté minced garlic and grated ginger until fragrant.
3. Add chopped vegetables and stir-fry until tender-crisp.
4. Stir in cooked quinoa.
5. Add soy sauce to taste.
6. Garnish with sliced green onions and sesame seeds.
7. Toss gently to combine.
8. Serve this Quinoa and Vegetable Stir-Fry for a colorful and nutritious meal.

Nutritional Information:
Calories: 280 | *Protein:* 10g | *Carbohydrates:* 40g | *Fat:* 8g | *Fiber:* 6g

Grilled Turkey Burgers with Sweet Potato Fries

Intro: Fire up the grill for Grilled Turkey Burgers with Sweet Potato Fries. These lean and flavorful turkey burgers are paired with crispy sweet potato fries, creating a satisfying and wholesome meal perfect for a barbecue.

Total Prep Time: 40 minutes

Ingredients:

Turkey Burgers:
- Ground turkey
- Onion, finely chopped
- Worcestershire sauce
- Dijon mustard
- Salt and pepper to taste

Sweet Potato Fries:
- Sweet potatoes, cut into fries
- Olive oil
- Paprika
- Garlic powder
- Salt and pepper to taste

Instructions:

Turkey Burgers:
1. In a bowl, mix ground turkey, chopped onion, Worcestershire sauce, Dijon mustard, salt, and pepper.
2. Form into burger patties.
3. Grill until fully cooked.

Sweet Potato Fries:
1. Preheat the oven to 400°F (200°C).
2. Toss sweet potato fries with olive oil, paprika, garlic powder, salt, and pepper.
3. Bake until fries are golden and crispy.
4. Serve Grilled Turkey Burgers with Sweet Potato Fries for a delicious and balanced meal.

Nutritional Information:
Calories: 350 | *Protein:* 25g | *Carbohydrates:* 30g | *Fat:* 15g | *Fiber:* 6g

Stuffed Portobello Mushrooms with Quinoa

Intro: Elevate your mushroom experience with Stuffed Portobello Mushrooms with Quinoa. These hearty and savory mushrooms are filled with a flavorful quinoa stuffing, creating a satisfying and nutritious dish.
Total Prep Time: 35 minutes

Ingredients:
- Portobello mushrooms, cleaned and stems removed
- Quinoa, cooked
- Spinach, chopped
- Feta cheese, crumbled
- Cherry tomatoes, diced
- Balsamic glaze
- Olive oil
- Salt and pepper to taste

Instructions:
1. Preheat the oven to 375°F (190°C).
2. Brush portobello mushrooms with olive oil and season with salt and pepper.
3. In a bowl, mix cooked quinoa, chopped spinach, crumbled feta, and diced cherry tomatoes.
4. Spoon the quinoa mixture into the portobello mushrooms.
5. Bake for 20-25 minutes or until mushrooms are tender.
6. Drizzle with balsamic glaze before serving.

7. Enjoy these Stuffed Portobello Mushrooms with Quinoa as a satisfying and flavorful meal.

Nutritional Information:

Calories: 280 | *Protein:* 12g | *Carbohydrates:* 35g | *Fat:* 10g | *Fiber:* 8g

Chicken and Broccoli Stir-Fry

Intro: Whip up a quick and delicious meal with Chicken and Broccoli Stir-Fry. This classic stir-fry features tender chicken, crisp broccoli, and a flavorful sauce, making it a go-to recipe for busy nights.

Total Prep Time: 25 minutes

Ingredients:
- Chicken breasts, thinly sliced
- Broccoli florets
- Soy sauce
- Hoisin sauce
- Sesame oil
- Garlic, minced
- Ginger, grated
- Red pepper flakes (optional)
- Green onions, sliced
- Cooked rice for serving

Instructions:
1. In a wok or large skillet, heat sesame oil.
2. Sauté minced garlic, grated ginger, and red pepper flakes if desired.
3. Add sliced chicken and cook until browned.
4. Add broccoli florets and stir-fry until tender-crisp.

5. In a bowl, mix soy sauce and hoisin sauce. Pour over the chicken and broccoli.
6. Toss until everything is coated in the sauce.
7. Garnish with sliced green onions.
8. Serve this Chicken and Broccoli Stir-Fry over cooked rice for a quick and tasty meal.

Nutritional Information:
Calories: 320 | *Protein:* 25g | *Carbohydrates:* 30g | *Fat:* 12g | *Fiber:* 5g

Roasted Vegetable and Lentil Casserole

Intro: Dive into a wholesome and hearty Roasted Vegetable and Lentil Casserole. This comforting dish combines roasted vegetables, nutritious lentils, and a savory tomato sauce, creating a flavorful and satisfying casserole.

Total Prep Time: 45 minutes

Ingredients:
- Mixed vegetables (zucchini, bell peppers, carrots), chopped
- Lentils, cooked
- Onion, finely chopped
- Garlic, minced
- Tomato sauce
- Italian seasoning
- Mozzarella cheese, shredded
- Olive oil
- Salt and pepper to taste

Instructions:
1. Preheat the oven to 375°F (190°C).

2. Toss chopped vegetables with olive oil, salt, and pepper.
3. Roast in the oven until vegetables are tender.
4. In a skillet, sauté chopped onion and minced garlic until softened.
5. Add cooked lentils, tomato sauce, and Italian seasoning. Cook for a few minutes.
6. In a casserole dish, layer roasted vegetables, lentil mixture, and shredded mozzarella.
7. Repeat layers until the dish is filled.
8. Bake for 20-25 minutes or until the cheese is melted and bubbly.
9. Serve this Roasted Vegetable and Lentil Casserole for a wholesome and flavorful dinner.

Nutritional Information:

Calories: 300 | *Protein:* 15g | *Carbohydrates:* 35g | *Fat:* 12g | *Fiber:* 10g

Baked Salmon with Lemon and Herbs

Intro: Indulge in the delicate flavors of the sea with Baked Salmon with Lemon and Herbs. This elegant dish features succulent salmon fillets seasoned with fresh herbs and zesty lemon, baked to perfection for a light and nutritious meal.

Total Prep Time: 30 minutes

Ingredients:
- Salmon fillets
- Fresh dill, chopped
- Fresh parsley, chopped
- Lemon zest
- Garlic, minced

- Olive oil
- Lemon slices
- Salt and pepper to taste

Instructions:
1. Preheat the oven to 400°F (200°C).
2. Place salmon fillets on a baking sheet.
3. In a bowl, mix chopped dill, chopped parsley, lemon zest, minced garlic, and olive oil.
4. Spread the herb mixture over the salmon fillets.
5. Season with salt and pepper.
6. Place lemon slices on top.
7. Bake for 15-20 minutes or until the salmon is cooked through.
8. Serve this Baked Salmon with Lemon and Herbs for a sophisticated and flavorful dinner.

Nutritional Information:
Calories: 320 | *Protein:* 30g | *Carbohydrates:* 2g | *Fat:* 22g | *Fiber:* 1g

Spaghetti Squash Primavera

Intro: Embrace a low-carb twist on a classic with Spaghetti Squash Primavera. This dish features roasted spaghetti squash strands tossed with a medley of vibrant vegetables and a light tomato sauce for a satisfying and healthy alternative to traditional pasta.

Total Prep Time: 50 minutes

Ingredients:
- 1 spaghetti squash, halved and seeds removed
- Olive oil
- Salt and pepper to taste

- Cherry tomatoes, halved
- Zucchini, sliced
- Bell peppers, sliced
- Garlic, minced
- Tomato sauce
- Fresh basil, chopped
- Parmesan cheese for topping

Instructions:
1. Preheat the oven to 400°F (200°C).
2. Drizzle spaghetti squash halves with olive oil and season with salt and pepper.
3. Roast for 40-45 minutes or until the squash is fork-tender.
4. Meanwhile, in a skillet, sauté minced garlic until fragrant.
5. Add cherry tomatoes, zucchini, and bell peppers. Cook until vegetables are tender.
6. Stir in tomato sauce and fresh basil.
7. Scrape the spaghetti squash with a fork to create strands.
8. Toss the squash strands with the vegetable and tomato mixture.
9. Serve Spaghetti Squash Primavera topped with Parmesan cheese for a light and flavorful meal.

Nutritional Information:
Calories: 220 | *Protein:* 8g | *Carbohydrates:* 40g | *Fat:* 8g | *Fiber:* 10g

Turkey and Spinach Meatballs with Zucchini Noodles

Intro: Dive into a lighter version of the classic with Turkey and Spinach Meatballs with Zucchini Noodles. These tender meatballs are paired with fresh zucchini noodles and a flavorful tomato sauce for a nutritious and satisfying meal.

Total Prep Time: 40 minutes

Ingredients:
Turkey and Spinach Meatballs:
- Ground turkey
- Spinach, chopped
- Onion, finely chopped
- Garlic, minced
- Egg
- Bread crumbs
- Italian seasoning
- Salt and pepper to taste

Zucchini Noodles:
- Zucchini, spiralized into noodles
- Olive oil
- Tomato sauce
- Fresh basil, chopped
- Parmesan cheese for topping

Instructions:
Turkey and Spinach Meatballs:
1. Preheat the oven to 375°F (190°C).
2. In a bowl, mix ground turkey, chopped spinach, chopped onion, minced garlic, egg, bread crumbs, Italian seasoning, salt, and pepper.

3. Form into meatballs and place on a baking sheet.
4. Bake for 20-25 minutes or until meatballs are cooked through.

Zucchini Noodles:
1. In a skillet, heat olive oil.
2. Sauté spiralized zucchini until just tender.
3. Pour tomato sauce over the zucchini noodles.
4. Add chopped fresh basil.
5. Serve Turkey and Spinach Meatballs over Zucchini Noodles topped with Parmesan cheese for a flavorful and light dinner.

Nutritional Information:

Calories: 300 | *Protein:* 25g | *Carbohydrates:* 20g | *Fat:* 15g | *Fiber:* 5g

Eggplant and Chickpea Tagine

Intro: Transport your taste buds to Morocco with Eggplant and Chickpea Tagine. This aromatic and hearty dish features tender eggplant, protein-packed chickpeas, and a flavorful blend of spices for a satisfying and exotic culinary experience.

Total Prep Time: 45 minutes

Ingredients:
- Eggplant, diced
- Chickpeas, cooked
- Onion, finely chopped
- Garlic, minced
- Tomatoes, diced
- Vegetable broth
- Ground cumin

- Ground coriander
- Smoked paprika
- Cinnamon
- Fresh cilantro, chopped
- Lemon wedges for serving
- Cooked couscous or rice for serving

Instructions:
1. In a large pot or tagine, sauté chopped onion and minced garlic until softened.
2. Add diced eggplant and cook until it begins to soften.
3. Stir in diced tomatoes, cooked chickpeas, vegetable broth, ground cumin, ground coriander, smoked paprika, and a pinch of cinnamon.
4. Simmer the tagine over medium heat for 25-30 minutes, allowing the flavors to meld and the vegetables to become tender.
5. Adjust seasoning if needed.
6. Sprinkle chopped fresh cilantro over the tagine.
7. Serve the Eggplant and Chickpea Tagine over cooked couscous or rice.
8. Accompany with lemon wedges for a burst of citrus flavor.

Nutritional Information:
Calories: 280 | *Protein:* 10g | *Carbohydrates:* 45g | *Fat:* 8g | *Fiber:* 12g

Lemon Herb Roasted Chicken

Intro: Elevate your dinner table with the delightful flavors of Lemon Herb Roasted Chicken. This classic roasted chicken recipe features a blend of aromatic herbs, zesty lemon, and tender chicken for a comforting and flavorful main course.

Total Prep Time: 1 hour

Ingredients:

- Whole chicken
- Fresh rosemary, chopped
- Fresh thyme, chopped
- Fresh parsley, chopped
- Lemon, sliced
- Garlic, minced
- Olive oil
- Salt and pepper to taste

Instructions:

1. Preheat the oven to 375°F (190°C).
2. Rinse the chicken and pat it dry with paper towels.
3. In a bowl, mix chopped rosemary, thyme, parsley, minced garlic, and olive oil.
4. Rub the herb mixture over the chicken, ensuring even coverage.
5. Season the chicken with salt and pepper.
6. Place lemon slices inside the chicken cavity.
7. Tie the chicken legs together with kitchen twine.
8. Roast in the oven for approximately 1 hour or until the internal temperature reaches 165°F (74°C).
9. Allow the chicken to rest for 10 minutes before carving.

Nutritional Information:

Calories: 300 | *Protein:* 25g | *Carbohydrates:* 2g | *Fat:* 20g | *Fiber:* 1g

Quinoa and Black Bean Bowl

Intro: Create a protein-packed and satisfying meal with the Quinoa and Black Bean Bowl. This wholesome bowl features fluffy quinoa, hearty black beans, and a medley of fresh vegetables, offering a nutritious and delicious dining experience.

Total Prep Time: 30 minutes

Ingredients:
- 1 cup quinoa, cooked
- Black beans, cooked and drained
- Corn kernels (fresh or frozen)
- Cherry tomatoes, halved
- Avocado, diced
- Red onion, finely chopped
- Cilantro, chopped
- Lime juice
- Olive oil
- Salt and pepper to taste

Instructions:
1. In a bowl, assemble cooked quinoa, black beans, corn, cherry tomatoes, diced avocado, chopped red onion, and cilantro.
2. In a small bowl, whisk together lime juice, olive oil, salt, and pepper.
3. Drizzle the dressing over the quinoa and black bean mixture.
4. Toss gently to combine.
5. Serve this Quinoa and Black Bean Bowl as a nourishing and flavorful meal.

Nutritional Information:

Calories: 320 | *Protein:* 15g | *Carbohydrates:* 50g | *Fat:* 10g | *Fiber:* 12g

Sweet Potato and Kale Hash

Intro: Start your day with the nutritious and flavorful Sweet Potato and Kale Hash. This hearty breakfast dish combines sweet potatoes, kale, and savory seasonings for a satisfying and wholesome way to kick off your morning.

Total Prep Time: 35 minutes

Ingredients:
- Sweet potatoes, peeled and diced
- Kale, chopped
- Onion, finely chopped
- Garlic, minced
- Olive oil
- Smoked paprika
- Cumin
- Salt and pepper to taste
- Poached eggs for serving (optional)

Instructions:
1. In a skillet, heat olive oil.
2. Sauté chopped onion and minced garlic until softened.
3. Add diced sweet potatoes and cook until they begin to brown.
4. Stir in chopped kale and continue cooking until kale wilts.
5. Season with smoked paprika, cumin, salt, and pepper.

6. Continue cooking until sweet potatoes are tender and kale is crispy.
7. Optional: Serve the Sweet Potato and Kale Hash with poached eggs on top for added protein.
8. Enjoy this flavorful and nutrient-rich breakfast.

Nutritional Information:

Calories: 250 | *Protein:* 6g | *Carbohydrates:* 40g | *Fat:* 8g | *Fiber:* 8g

Shrimp and Vegetable Skewers

Intro: Fire up the grill for Shrimp and Vegetable Skewers, a delightful and light option for your summer gatherings. These skewers feature succulent shrimp, colorful vegetables, and a zesty marinade, creating a flavorful and healthy dish.

Total Prep Time: 25 minutes

Ingredients:

- Shrimp, peeled and deveined
- Cherry tomatoes
- Bell peppers, cut into chunks
- Red onion, cut into wedges
- Zucchini, sliced
- Olive oil
- Lemon juice
- Garlic, minced
- Fresh parsley, chopped
- Salt and pepper to taste

Instructions:

1. Preheat the grill or grill pan.

2. In a bowl, mix olive oil, lemon juice, minced garlic, chopped fresh parsley, salt, and pepper.
3. Thread shrimp, cherry tomatoes, bell peppers, red onion, and zucchini onto skewers.
4. Brush the skewers with the olive oil and lemon marinade.
5. Grill the skewers for 4-5 minutes per side or until the shrimp is opaque.
6. Serve these Shrimp and Vegetable Skewers for a delightful and healthy barbecue option.

Nutritional Information:
Calories: 280 | *Protein:* 20g | *Carbohydrates:* 15g | *Fat:* 15g | *Fiber:* 4g

Cauliflower Fried Rice with Tofu

Intro: Enjoy a lighter take on a classic with Cauliflower Fried Rice with Tofu. This low-carb and nutritious dish feature riced cauliflower, tofu, and a colorful array of vegetables, creating a satisfying and flavorful alternative to traditional fried rice.

Total Prep Time: 30 minutes

Ingredients:
- Cauliflower, riced
- Extra-firm tofu, pressed and cubed
- Carrots, diced
- Peas
- Corn kernels (fresh or frozen)
- Scallions, sliced
- Soy sauce
- Sesame oil
- Ginger, grated

- Garlic, minced
- Olive oil
- Sesame seeds for topping

Instructions:
1. In a large skillet or wok, heat olive oil.
2. Add cubed tofu and cook until golden brown on all sides.
3. Push tofu to one side of the skillet and add grated ginger and minced garlic. Sauté until fragrant.
4. Add diced carrots, peas, and corn. Stir-fry until vegetables are tender.
5. Push the vegetables to the side and add riced cauliflower to the skillet.
6. Pour soy sauce and sesame oil over the cauliflower and toss to combine with the vegetables.
7. Mix in sliced scallions and cooked tofu.
8. Cook for an additional 5-7 minutes until the cauliflower is cooked through.
9. Serve this Cauliflower Fried Rice with Tofu topped with sesame seeds for a delicious and guilt-free meal.

Nutritional Information:
Calories: 250 | *Protein:* 15g | *Carbohydrates:* 20g | *Fat:* 12g | *Fiber:* 8g

Turkey and Quinoa Stuffed Acorn Squash

Intro: Embrace the flavors of fall with Turkey and Quinoa Stuffed Acorn Squash. This hearty and nutritious dish features a savory filling of ground turkey, quinoa, and aromatic spices, nestled within roasted acorn squash halves.

Total Prep Time: 1 hour

Ingredients:
- Acorn squash, halved and seeds removed
- Ground turkey
- Quinoa, cooked
- Onion, finely chopped
- Garlic, minced
- Cranberries, dried
- Pecans, chopped
- Sage, chopped
- Olive oil
- Salt and pepper to taste

Instructions:
1. Preheat the oven to 375°F (190°C).
2. Place acorn squash halves on a baking sheet.
3. Drizzle with olive oil and season with salt and pepper.
4. Roast for 30-40 minutes or until squash is tender.
5. In a skillet, sauté chopped onion and minced garlic until softened.
6. Add ground turkey and cook until browned.
7. Stir in cooked quinoa, dried cranberries, chopped pecans, and sage.
8. Spoon the turkey and quinoa mixture into the roasted acorn squash halves.
9. Bake for an additional 15-20 minutes.
10. Serve Turkey and Quinoa Stuffed Acorn Squash for a comforting and autumn-inspired meal.

Nutritional Information:
Calories: 350 | *Protein:* 25g | *Carbohydrates:* 30g | *Fat:* 15g | *Fiber:* 8g

Mediterranean Baked Cod

Intro: Transport your taste buds to the shores of the Mediterranean with this flavorful Mediterranean Baked Cod. This light and heart-healthy dish feature cod fillets seasoned with a blend of Mediterranean herbs, roasted tomatoes, and Kalamata olives.
Total Prep Time: 25 minutes

Ingredients:
- Cod fillets
- Cherry tomatoes, halved
- Kalamata olives, pitted and sliced
- Fresh oregano, chopped
- Fresh parsley, chopped
- Garlic, minced
- Lemon, sliced
- Olive oil
- Salt and pepper to taste

Instructions:
1. Preheat the oven to 375°F (190°C).
2. Place cod fillets in a baking dish.
3. Surround the cod with halved cherry tomatoes and sliced Kalamata olives.
4. In a bowl, mix chopped oregano, chopped parsley, minced garlic, and olive oil.
5. Drizzle the herb mixture over the cod fillets.
6. Season with salt and pepper.
7. Place lemon slices on top.
8. Bake for 15-20 minutes or until the cod is cooked through.
9. Serve this Mediterranean Baked Cod with a side of quinoa or couscous for a light and flavorful meal.

Nutritional Information:
Calories: 280 | *Protein:* 30g | *Carbohydrates:* 8g | *Fat:* 15g | *Fiber:* 2g

Lentil and Vegetable Curry

Intro: Dive into a bowl of comfort with Lentil and Vegetable Curry. This vegetarian delight features protein-rich lentils, an array of colorful vegetables, and a fragrant blend of curry spices, creating a hearty and satisfying dish.

Total Prep Time: 40 minutes

Ingredients:
- Lentils, cooked
- Onion, finely chopped
- Carrots, diced
- Bell peppers, diced
- Zucchini, diced
- Coconut milk
- Tomato sauce
- Curry powder
- Cumin
- Coriander
- Turmeric
- Garlic, minced
- Ginger, grated
- Olive oil
- Fresh cilantro, chopped
- Cooked rice for serving

Instructions:
1. In a large pot, sauté chopped onion, minced garlic, and grated ginger in olive oil until softened.

2. Add diced carrots, bell peppers, and zucchini. Cook until vegetables begin to soften.
3. Stir in cooked lentils, coconut milk, and tomato sauce.
4. Add curry powder, cumin, coriander, turmeric, and salt to taste.
5. Simmer the curry for 20-25 minutes, allowing the flavors to meld.
6. Adjust seasoning if needed.
7. Serve Lentil and Vegetable Curry over cooked rice.
8. Garnish with chopped fresh cilantro.
9. Enjoy this comforting and nutritious curry.

Nutritional Information:

Calories: 300 | *Protein:* 15g | *Carbohydrates:* 40g | *Fat:* 10g | *Fiber:* 12g

Chicken and Asparagus Stir-Fry

Intro: Whip up a quick and flavorful Chicken and Asparagus Stir-Fry for a delicious and nutritious meal. This stir-fry features tender chicken, crisp asparagus, and a savory sauce that comes together in no time.

Total Prep Time: 30 minutes

Ingredients:
- Chicken breasts, thinly sliced
- Asparagus spears, trimmed and cut into pieces
- Soy sauce
- Hoisin sauce
- Sesame oil
- Garlic, minced
- Ginger, grated
- Red pepper flakes (optional)

- Green onions, sliced
- Cooked brown rice for serving

Instructions:
1. In a wok or large skillet, heat sesame oil.
2. Sauté minced garlic, grated ginger, and red pepper flakes if desired.
3. Add sliced chicken and cook until browned.
4. Add asparagus pieces and stir-fry until they are tender-crisp.
5. In a bowl, mix soy sauce and hoisin sauce. Pour over the chicken and asparagus.
6. Toss until everything is coated in the sauce.
7. Garnish with sliced green onions.
8. Serve this Chicken and Asparagus Stir-Fry over cooked brown rice for a quick and tasty meal.

Nutritional Information:
Calories: 320 | *Protein:* 25g | *Carbohydrates:* 30g | *Fat:* 12g | *Fiber:* 5g

Pesto Zoodles with Cherry Tomatoes

Intro: Indulge in a light and flavorful meal with Pesto Zoodles with Cherry Tomatoes. This low-carb dish features spiralized zucchini noodles tossed in vibrant pesto and topped with burst cherry tomatoes for a refreshing and satisfying experience.

Total Prep Time: 20 minutes

Ingredients:
- Zucchini, spiralized into noodles
- Cherry tomatoes, halved
- Pesto sauce

- Parmesan cheese, grated
- Pine nuts for topping
- Olive oil
- Salt and pepper to taste

Instructions:
1. In a large skillet, heat olive oil.
2. Add spiralized zucchini noodles and cook for 2-3 minutes until just tender.
3. Toss in cherry tomatoes and cook for an additional 2 minutes.
4. Stir in pesto sauce and coat the zoodles and tomatoes evenly.
5. Season with salt and pepper to taste.
6. Transfer to a serving dish.
7. Sprinkle grated Parmesan cheese and pine nuts over the top.
8. Serve these Pesto Zoodles with Cherry Tomatoes as a light and delightful meal.

Nutritional Information:
Calories: 220 | *Protein:* 6g | *Carbohydrates:* 15g | *Fat:* 18g | *Fiber:* 4g

Baked Chicken with Brussels Sprouts

Intro: Enjoy a one-pan wonder with Baked Chicken with Brussels Sprouts. This easy and wholesome dish features seasoned chicken thighs baked to perfection alongside roasted Brussels sprouts, creating a fuss-free and flavorful meal.

Total Prep Time: 40 minutes

Ingredients:

- Chicken thighs, bone-in and skin-on
- Brussels sprouts, trimmed and halved
- Garlic, minced
- Lemon zest
- Paprika
- Thyme, dried
- Olive oil
- Salt and pepper to taste

Instructions:

1. Preheat the oven to 400°F (200°C).
2. In a bowl, mix minced garlic, lemon zest, paprika, dried thyme, olive oil, salt, and pepper.
3. Place chicken thighs on a baking sheet.
4. Toss Brussels sprouts in the same bowl with the seasoning mixture.
5. Arrange Brussels sprouts around the chicken thighs.
6. Bake for 25-30 minutes or until the chicken is cooked through and Brussels sprouts are golden and crispy.
7. Serve this Baked Chicken with Brussels Sprouts for a simple and wholesome dinner.

Nutritional Information:

Calories: 350 | *Protein:* 30g | *Carbohydrates:* 10g | *Fat:* 22g | *Fiber:* 4g

Spinach and Feta Stuffed Chicken Breast

Intro: Elevate your chicken dinner with Spinach and Feta Stuffed Chicken Breast. This elegant dish features juicy chicken breasts stuffed with a flavorful mixture of spinach and feta, creating a delightful and impressive main course.

Total Prep Time: 45 minutes

Ingredients:

- Chicken breasts, boneless and skinless
- Fresh spinach, chopped
- Feta cheese, crumbled
- Garlic, minced
- Olive oil
- Lemon juice
- Dill, chopped
- Salt and pepper to taste

Instructions:

1. Preheat the oven to 375°F (190°C).
2. In a skillet, sauté chopped spinach and minced garlic in olive oil until wilted.
3. Remove from heat and stir in crumbled feta, lemon juice, chopped dill, salt, and pepper.
4. Butterfly the chicken breasts and stuff each with the spinach and feta mixture.
5. Secure the chicken breasts with toothpicks.
6. Place the stuffed chicken breasts in a baking dish.
7. Bake for 25-30 minutes or until the chicken is cooked through.
8. Serve this Spinach and Feta Stuffed Chicken Breast for an impressive and flavorful dinner.

Nutritional Information:

Calories: 320 | *Protein:* 35g | *Carbohydrates:* 4g | *Fat:* 18g | *Fiber:* 2g

Quinoa and Vegetable Stuffed Mushrooms

Intro: Elevate your appetizer game with Quinoa and Vegetable Stuffed Mushrooms. These bite-sized delights feature a savory filling of quinoa, colorful vegetables, and melted cheese, creating a crowd-pleasing and nutritious snack.

Total Prep Time: 35 minutes

Ingredients:
- Large mushrooms, cleaned and stems removed
- Quinoa, cooked
- Red bell pepper, finely diced
- Zucchini, finely diced
- Onion, finely diced
- Garlic, minced
- Mozzarella cheese, shredded
- Parmesan cheese, grated
- Olive oil
- Italian seasoning
- Salt and pepper to taste

Instructions:
1. Preheat the oven to 375°F (190°C).
2. Brush the mushroom caps with olive oil and place them on a baking sheet.
3. In a skillet, sauté diced onion and minced garlic until softened.
4. Add diced red bell pepper and zucchini. Cook until vegetables are tender.
5. Stir in cooked quinoa and Italian seasoning. Season with salt and pepper.
6. Spoon the quinoa and vegetable mixture into each mushroom cap.

7. Top with shredded mozzarella and grated Parmesan cheese.
8. Bake for 15-20 minutes or until the mushrooms are tender and the cheese is melted and golden.
9. Serve these Quinoa and Vegetable Stuffed Mushrooms as a delightful appetizer or side dish.

Nutritional Information:

Calories: 180 | *Protein:* 8g | *Carbohydrates:* 20g | *Fat:* 8g | *Fiber:* 4g

Teriyaki Salmon with Brown Rice

Intro: Savor the delicate flavors of Teriyaki Salmon with Brown Rice. This wholesome dish features succulent salmon fillets glazed with a sweet and savory teriyaki sauce, served over nutty brown rice for a balanced and satisfying meal.

Total Prep Time: 30 minutes

Ingredients:
- Salmon fillets
- Brown rice, cooked
- Teriyaki sauce
- Soy sauce
- Mirin
- Brown sugar
- Garlic, minced
- Ginger, grated
- Green onions, sliced
- Sesame seeds for topping

Instructions:

1. In a bowl, mix teriyaki sauce, soy sauce, mirin, minced garlic, and grated ginger to create the teriyaki glaze.
2. Place salmon fillets in a baking dish and brush them with the teriyaki glaze.
3. Bake in the oven at 375°F (190°C) for 15-20 minutes or until the salmon is cooked through.
4. While the salmon is baking, prepare brown rice according to package instructions.
5. Serve the Teriyaki Salmon over a bed of brown rice.
6. Drizzle with additional teriyaki glaze.
7. Garnish with sliced green onions and sesame seeds.
8. Enjoy this Teriyaki Salmon with Brown Rice for a delicious and nourishing dinner.

Nutritional Information:

Calories: 350 | *Protein:* 25g | *Carbohydrates:* 30g | *Fat:* 15g | *Fiber:* 3g

Stuffed Cabbage Rolls with Turkey and Quinoa

Intro: Delight in the comfort of Stuffed Cabbage Rolls with Turkey and Quinoa. This wholesome dish features cabbage leaves filled with a savory mixture of ground turkey, quinoa, and aromatic spices, all simmered in a flavorful tomato sauce.

Total Prep Time: 1 hour and 15 minutes

Ingredients:

- Cabbage leaves, blanched
- Ground turkey
- Quinoa, cooked

- Onion, finely chopped
- Garlic, minced
- Tomato sauce
- Diced tomatoes
- Paprika
- Thyme, dried
- Bay leaves
- Olive oil
- Salt and pepper to taste

Instructions:
1. Preheat the oven to 375°F (190°C).
2. In a skillet, sauté chopped onion and minced garlic in olive oil until softened.
3. Add ground turkey and cook until browned.
4. Stir in cooked quinoa, diced tomatoes, paprika, dried thyme, salt, and pepper.
5. Remove the tough center stalk from each blanched cabbage leaf.
6. Place a portion of the turkey and quinoa mixture onto each cabbage leaf and roll them up.
7. Place the cabbage rolls in a baking dish.
8. In a bowl, mix tomato sauce and bay leaves. Pour the sauce over the cabbage rolls.
9. Cover the baking dish with foil and bake for 40-45 minutes.
10. Serve these Stuffed Cabbage Rolls with Turkey and Quinoa for a comforting and wholesome dinner.

Nutritional Information:
Calories: 280 | *Protein:* 20g | *Carbohydrates:* 30g | *Fat:* 10g | *Fiber:* 6g